BLADDER

Therapies For Overactive Bladder And UTI Prevention

Achieve Bladder Bliss With Therapies Addressing Overactive Bladder Issues And Promoting Urinary Tract Health

DR. BRIDGET PROMISE

Table of Contents

CHAPTER ONE 4

   Introduction 4

   Exploring The Bladder: A Brief 5

   Frequent Aetiologies Of Overactive..............7

   Signs And Symptoms: Determining Overactive Bladder..10

CHAPTER TWO 12

   The Effects Of Bladder Overactivity On Everyday Life..12

   Medical Strategies For The Management Of Overactive Bladder 14

   Dietary Considerations: Beneficial And Adverse Foods...19

CHAPTER THREE..22

   Hydration Practices: Maximizing Water Consumption..22

   Natural Remedies For The Relief Of.............29

   Supplements And Herbal 30

CHAPTER FOUR 33

   Mind-Body Techniques For 33

   Developing An Understanding Of 35

Keeping The Urinary Tract Healthy 37

CHAPTER FIVE 41

Hygiene Practices To Prevent Utis 41

Efficient Antibiotics For The 44

Bladder-Safe Meal Plans And 46

CHAPTER SIX 50

Integrating Holistic Healing 50

Ensuring Sustained Bladder 52

In Summary, The Attainment Of 54

CHAPTER ONE

Introduction

Overactive bladder (OAB) is a widely prevalent medical condition that has a profound impact on the daily lives and quality of life of millions of individuals worldwide.

This pathological state is distinguished by an abrupt, involuntary spasm of the bladder muscles, resulting in an intense urge to defecate despite the bladder not being filled.

This extensive investigation will cover every aspect of the overactive bladder, including its physiological intricacies, prevalent etiology, manifestations, and the practical implications it poses. Furthermore, an examination of the medical interventions utilized in the treatment of overactive bladder will be included.

Exploring The Bladder: A Brief Introduction

Before one can fully grasp the complexities of an overactive bladder, it is vital to acquire a fundamental understanding of the bladder's typical operation. The bladder is a pelvic-regional muscular organ that is essential for the storage and discharge of urine. Anatomically, the bladder muscles maintain a state of relaxation during the progressive filtration of urine.

Upon the bladder reaching its maximum capacity, neural signals are transmitted to the brain, inducing an intentional decision to excrete. Throughout this process, the muscles encircling the urethra relax, and the muscles in the bladder contract, allowing the urine to seep out.

This coordination between the brain and the muscles of the bladder, however, is disrupted in those with overactive bladder. The involuntary contraction of the bladder muscles induces an urgent urination response, which frequently results in frequent and occasionally unplanned visits to the restroom.

This disturbance in the delicate equilibrium of muscle coordination is the fundamental cause of overactive bladder syndrome.

Frequent Aetiologies Of Overactive Bladder

A variety of factors can contribute to overactive bladder; therefore, it is vital to identify these triggers to conduct effective management. Age is a significant factor, as the muscular strength of the bladder gradually declines with age, increasing the likelihood of involuntary contractions. Overactivity may also result from neurological disorders such as Parkinson's disease or multiple sclerosis, which disrupt the normal function of the bladder muscles.

Infections of the urinary tract (UTIs) and stones in the bladder can also irritate the bladder, which can exacerbate the symptoms of overactive bladder. Specific pharmaceuticals, such as diuretics, have the potential to stimulate urinary output, thereby exacerbating the need to evacuate. Additionally, certain lifestyle choices, including the consumption of piquant foods and excessive caffeine, may worsen symptoms in certain individuals.

It is of the utmost importance to identify the underlying cause of overactive bladder to develop an effective treatment strategy, as addressing these factors can substantially enhance the condition's management.

Signs And Symptoms: Determining Overactive Bladder

It is critical to identify the symptoms of an overactive bladder to seek medical attention promptly. An intense, sudden urge to excrete is the defining characteristic; this is frequently accompanied by the dread of missing the restroom.

Additionally, some cases of urinary incontinence (inability to control urine discharge) and increased frequency of urination (waking up multiple times during the night to use the restroom) may be experienced by those with overactive bladder.

It is crucial to acknowledge that although nocturnal urgency or nocturia (urination at night) may not invariably signify an overactive bladder, chronic and disruptive symptoms require medical attention.

It is imperative to seek the guidance of a healthcare professional to obtain an accurate diagnosis, as they possess the ability to differentiate overactive bladder from other urinary disorders and provide suitable treatment recommendations.

CHAPTER TWO

The Effects Of Bladder Overactivity On Everyday Life

The ramifications of an overactive bladder transcend the domain of the corporeal, exerting a substantial influence on an individual's daily functioning and general state of health.

Constantly rescheduling activities to accommodate the availability of restrooms can inhibit social interactions and result in feelings of humiliation and isolation. A great number of people may avoid lengthy excursions or activities out of concern for the unpredictability of their symptoms.

An overactive bladder has an immense emotional toll that cannot be exaggerated. Frequent companions of anxiety and tension are the anticipation of the next impulse, thereby establishing a recurring pattern that may worsen symptoms.

Nocturia-related sleep disruptions may result in cognitive decline and fatigue, which may hurt work performance and overall productivity.

In addition to medical interventions, psychological and

lifestyle modifications are required to mitigate the daily effects of overactive bladder. By providing a forum for individuals to share their coping mechanisms and experiences, support groups and counseling can foster a sense of community and mutual understanding.

Medical Strategies For The Management Of Overactive Bladder

The management of overactive bladder frequently necessitates a comprehensive strategy that incorporates medical interventions, adjustments to one's lifestyle, and occasionally, surgical interventions. Medications that relax bladder muscles and ameliorate symptoms are frequently prescribed, including anticholinergics and beta-3 agonists. These medications inhibit the signals responsible for inducing involuntary contractions.

Behavioral therapies, such as pelvic floor exercises and bladder training, are essential elements in the management of overactive bladder.

Bladder training entails scheduling restroom visits to progressively extend the intervals between urinations, thereby facilitating the bladder's retraining to retain urine for extended durations. By fortifying the muscles responsible for urination, pelvic floor exercises enhance urinary control.

In cases where behavioral interventions and medication fail to be effective, advanced treatments like neuromodulation or Botox injections into the bladder muscles may be contemplated.

Surgical interventions aimed at augmenting bladder capacity or establishing a diversion for urinary storage may be advised in certain cases.

In summary, overactive bladder is an all-encompassing and intricate disorder that necessitates a holistic strategy for control. A holistic perspective is crucial for comprehending the normal functioning of the bladder, identifying prevalent causes, recognizing symptoms, and addressing the implications for daily life.

By integrating behavioral therapies and lifestyle modifications with medical interventions, individuals can be enabled to regain autonomy over their bladder function and experience increased satisfaction in their lives. Consistent communication with healthcare practitioners and the presence of a support system can be crucial in effectively managing the difficulties that arise from an overactive bladder.

Preserving optimal bladder health is of the utmost importance for one's overall health and quality of life. Developing an informed stance regarding bladder training, nutrition, hydration, and pelvic floor exercises, among other aspects, can significantly contribute to the maintenance of a healthy and resilient bladder.

Dietary Considerations: Beneficial And Adverse Foods

Bladder health may be significantly influenced by the nutrients we eat. Specific dietary decisions have the potential to either facilitate or impede urination. Maintaining dietary awareness is crucial to mitigate the potential for bladder-related complications.

1. Foods that assist:

• Consumption of Water-Rich Vegetables and Fruits: Including watermelon, cucumber, and celery in one's dietary regimen can promote urinary health and enhance overall hydration.

• Foods High in Fiber: Vegetables, whole grains, and legumes that are abundant in fiber aid in the maintenance of regular digestive movements, thereby averting constipation, which could potentially be a contributing factor to bladder complications.

2. Foods That Cause Damage:

Caffeine, which is present in specific beverages, coffee, and tea, functions as a diuretic by stimulating urine production and potentially causing irritation to the bladder.

- Citrus Fruits: Although citrus fruits are abundant in vitamin C, their acidic nature may irritate the bladder in certain individuals.

- Spicy Foods: The bladder membrane may be irritated by spices and spicy chiles, which may result in discomfort or a sense of urgency.

CHAPTER THREE

Hydration Practices: Maximizing Water Consumption

Sufficient hydration is an essential component of good health, and the maintenance of an ideal homeostasis is critical for proper bladder functioning. Although maintaining proper hydration is critical, it is equally imperative to exercise caution regarding the selection and quantity of liquids consumed.

1. Intake Guidelines for Water:

- Daily Water Consumption: Including all beverages and

dietary sources of water, the National Academies of Sciences, Engineering, and Medicine advise men to consume approximately 3.7 liters (125 ounces) and women 2.7 liters (91 ounces) of total water intake, respectively.

• Observe Urine Color: Adequate hydration is indicated by a pale yellow hue, whereas dehydration may be indicated by dark yellow or amber hues.

2. Optimal Methods of Hydration:

• Disperse Consumption: It is more beneficial to consume water in small quantities throughout the day rather than in large quantities all at once.

- Caffeinated and alcoholic beverages should be consumed in moderation to promote overall hydration, as they have the potential to function as diuretics.

Methods for Training the Bladder

The behavioral technique of bladder training is designed to increase bladder control and decrease urgency. Individuals who suffer from urinary incontinence or frequent urination frequently find it advantageous.

1. Prearranged Voiding:

One effective method of training the bladder is to schedule restroom breaks at consistent intervals, progressively extending the duration between discharges.

One effective method of resisting the impulse to urinate between scheduled times is to engage in the practice of deferring voiding for a few minutes at a time.

2. Alternate Voiding:

- Repeat the Bladder Emptying Process: Following urination, allow a brief interval before attempting to discharge once more. This technique may assist in achieving a more comprehensive bladder emptying.

3. Bladder Control Kegel Exercises: Pelvic Floor Exercises

By fortifying the pelvic floor muscles via Kegel exercises, bladder control can be effectively improved. The muscles that provide support for the bladder, urethra, and other pelvic organs are targeted by these exercises.

1. Palpating the Muscles of the Pelvic Floor:

• Muscle Identification: To isolate the pelvic floor muscles, endeavor to halt the midstream passage of urine. Kegel exercises target the muscles that are involved in this physical action.

2. Engaging in Kegel Exercises:

• Contract and Maintain: Maintain pressure on the pelvic floor muscles for three to five seconds.

• unwind and Release: Provide an equivalent amount of time for the muscles to unwind.

Aim to perform three sets of ten repetitions daily.

3. Performing Kegel Exercises daily:

- Establishing Routine Reminders: Integrate Kegel exercises into one's daily routine by linking them to recurring activities, such as flossing one's teeth or watching television commercials.

By incorporating lifestyle modifications into one's routine, one can proactively prevent and manage bladder-related complications. By implementing bladder training techniques, making dietary adjustments, maintaining proper hydration, and performing pelvic floor exercises, individuals can regain authority over their urinary health and experience enhanced daily comfort and self-assurance. It is recommended that individuals with persistent bladder issues seek the advice and support of healthcare professionals to receive individualized guidance and support that is specifically tailored to their requirements.

Natural Remedies For The Relief Of Overactive Bladder

Having an overactive bladder can present difficulties in daily life, affecting numerous facets. Relief can be obtained through natural therapies and modifications to one's lifestyle, which obviates the need for invasive treatments or medication. These methodologies comprise preventative measures, herbal remedies, and mind-body techniques, all of which contribute to the overall well-being of the bladder.

Supplements And Herbal Remedies For Bladder Health

Diverse cultures have utilized dietary supplements and herbs to promote bladder health and ameliorate the symptoms of overactive bladder for centuries. A noteworthy botanical specimen is Gosha-jinki-gan, an authentic

Japanese herbal formulation comprising Rehmannia Root and Japanese Silver Apricot, among other components. Research indicates that this herbal remedy has the potential to enhance bladder function and decrease urinary frequency.

Certain dietary supplements, alongside herbal remedies, contribute to the maintenance of optimal bladder health. One potential treatment for overactive bladder symptoms is pumpkin seed extract, which has demonstrated efficacy in improving prostate health in males and overall bladder function in females. Similarly, Cranberry Extract is widely recognized for its potential to inhibit urinary tract infections (UTIs), thus indirectly contributing to the management of overactive bladder.

When contemplating the use of herbal remedies and supplements, it is imperative to seek guidance from a healthcare professional to ascertain the appropriate dosage and verify the absence of any potential drug interactions with current medications.

CHAPTER FOUR
Mind-Body Techniques For Reducing Stress

Managing symptoms of overactive bladder is significantly aided by the mind-body connection, especially when tension exacerbates the condition. Engaging in routines such as yoga and meditation can have a beneficial effect on bladder function by alleviating tension and fostering relaxation.

Yoga, through its incorporation of deliberate breathing and mild motions, has the potential to enhance bodily awareness and fortify the pelvic muscles. Specific yoga positions, including Child's Pose and Bridge Pose, have the potential to provide relief to individuals experiencing overactive bladder through the activation of the pelvic floor muscles.

Conversely, engaging in meditation facilitates the development of mindfulness and the alleviation of anxiety. The implementation of stress management strategies, including the utilization of guided imagery and deep breathing exercises, may potentially alleviate the frequency and intensity of overactive bladder symptoms by promoting a more tranquil nervous system.

Developing An Understanding Of The Connection: Preventing Utis

UTIs of the urinary tract are a frequent cause of symptoms associated with overactive bladder. Comprehending the correlation between urinary tract infections and overactive bladder is critical for the successful management of the condition.

A bladder that is irritated by recurrent urinary tract infections may experience an increase in both the frequency and urgency of urination. Hydration is essential for preventing urinary tract infections because it aids in the elimination of pathogens from the urinary tract. A sufficient quantity of water consumed daily can reduce the risk of infection and dilute urine.

Furthermore, it is critical to maintain proper hygiene practices to avert the infiltration of pathogens into the urinary tract. This includes avoiding the use of aggravating feminine hygiene products, releasing the bladder before and following sexual activity, and cleaning from front to back.

Keeping The Urinary Tract Healthy

A comprehensive strategy for managing overactive bladder entails the preservation of urinary tract health as a whole. Self-care practices and straightforward adjustments to one's lifestyle can aid in the prevention of symptoms.

As part of the behavioral technique known as "Bladder Training," the interval between restroom trips is progressively extended. This method assists in retraining the bladder to retain urine for extended durations, thereby decreasing the frequency of impulses.

Additionally, dietary modifications have a substantial impact on urinary tract health. By avoiding bladder irritants like caffeine, piquant foods, and acidic fruits, symptoms of an overactive bladder can be reduced. Conversely, the inclusion of antioxidant-rich foods in one's diet, such as verdant greens and berries, may promote optimal bladder function.

Kegel exercises, also referred to as pelvic floor exercises, target and fortify the muscles responsible for regulating urinary flow. Engaging in these exercises consistently can enhance urinary control and alleviate the distress associated with overactive bladder.

In summary, natural remedies for alleviating overactive bladder comprise a diverse array of strategies, including preventative measures, mind-body practices, and botanical supplements and remedies.

By integrating these approaches into their daily routines, people can adopt a proactive stance to effectively manage their symptoms and enhance the overall health of their bladder. To ensure safety and efficacy, it is essential to consult with healthcare professionals before beginning a new treatment regimen.

CHAPTER FIVE

Hygiene Practices To Prevent Utis

Ensuring adequate sanitation is fundamental in the prevention of urinary tract infections (UTIs). A conduit connecting the bladder to the exterior of the body, the urethra, is a frequent entrance point for microorganisms.

Implementing sanitation practices that ensure the cleanliness of this area can substantially mitigate the likelihood of developing urinary tract infections (UTIs).

1. Maintaining adequate hydration aids in the elimination of

pathogens from the urinary tract. Aim to consume a minimum of eight glasses of water daily to stay hydrated.

2. Wipe Front to Back: Always wipe from front to back when using the restroom. By performing this uncomplicated procedure, the risk of pathogens entering the urethra from the anal region is reduced.

3. Regularly Empties Your Bladder: Avoid holding urine in for extended periods. Regular urination effectively prevents the proliferation of microorganisms within the bladder.

4. It is advisable for women to maintain proper feminine hygiene by selecting moderate, unscented cleansers to cleanse the genital area. Bruises and abrasive solvents should be avoided, as they can disturb the equilibrium of microorganisms.

5. Utilize Breathable Undergarments: Select cotton undergarments, which facilitate enhanced airflow and mitigate moisture, thereby establishing an environment that is less favorable for the proliferation of bacteria.

6. It is beneficial to void the bladder before and following

sexual activity to eliminate any pathogens that may have entered through the urethra.

Efficient Antibiotics For The Treatment Of Utis

Prompt and effective treatment is crucial to prevent the progression of a urinary tract infection to the kidneys. Antibiotics are frequently prescribed to eradicate the causative bacteria organisms. Prescribed antibiotics frequently consist of:

1. Nitrofurantoin, which is effective against a broad spectrum of bacteria, is frequently

prescribed for simple urinary tract infections.

2. The combination antibiotic Trimethoprim/Sulfamethoxazole (TMP/SMX) is efficacious against a range of bacterial infections, including urinary tract infections.

3. Reserved for the most severe cases, ciprofloxacin is an antibiotic with a broad spectrum of activity that is effective against a wide range of microorganisms.

Adherence to the prescribed course of antibiotics by a healthcare professional is of utmost importance, notwithstanding the resolution of symptoms before medication completion. Recurrence of the infection and development of antibiotic resistance may result from incomplete regimens of antibiotics.

Bladder-Safe Meal Plans And Recipes

A crucial factor in maintaining bladder health and preventing UTIs is dietary intake. Particular beverages and foods can aggravate the bladder, thereby exacerbating UTI symptoms. The integration of bladder-friendly meal plans and recipes can facilitate the prevention and management of urinary tract infections.

1. Maintaining sufficient hydration is essential for diluting urine and eliminating bacteria. Although water is the optimal option, caffeine-free medicinal beverages may also be consumed to enhance fluid consumption.

2. Cranberry Products May Prevent UTIs: Although the evidence is contradictory, several studies indicate that compounds in cranberries may inhibit bacterial adhesion to the bladder wall, thereby preventing UTIs. Supplements or unadulterated

cranberry juice should be consumed in moderation.

3. Opt for Whole Grains: Oats, brown rice, and quinoa are examples of whole grains that are abundant in fiber, which reduces the risk of urinary tract infections by regulating digestive movements and preventing constipation.

4. Incorporate Probiotics: Yogurt and other fermented foods contain probiotics, which promote a harmonious bacterial balance in the gastrointestinal tract and may indirectly enhance bladder health.

5. Caffeine and piquant foods can irritate the bladder and worsen

symptoms of a urinary tract infection; therefore, they should be restricted. When preparing meals, choose decaffeinated beverages and use less potent seasonings.

CHAPTER SIX
Integrating Holistic Healing Approaches

Holistic approaches to wellness incorporate lifestyle decisions that foster holistic well-being, thereby potentially exerting a beneficial influence on bladder health. These practices can improve the body's capacity to prevent and treat urinary tract infections.

1. Chronic tension compromises the integrity of the immune system, thereby increasing the body's vulnerability to infections. Stress management can be aided by yoga, meditation, and deep

breathing, among other techniques.

2. Engaging in regular physical activity not only aids in weight maintenance but also supports immune function, circulation, and resistance to urinary tract infections (UTIs).

3. Sufficient Sleep: Insufficient sleep can undermine the functionality of the immune system, thereby diminishing the body's capacity to combat infections. Aim for seven to nine hours of restful sleep per night.

4. Cessation of smoking is advised due to its potential to induce

chronic inflammation and undermine immune function. There are numerous health benefits associated with quitting smoking, including enhanced urinary health.

Ensuring Sustained Bladder Health

Sustaining bladder health necessitates continuous dedication and attention. Developing routines that encourage sustained urinary tract infection (UTI) prevention can aid in the prevention of UTIs and improve overall health.

1. It is advisable to establish a routine for check-ups with a healthcare provider to monitor and manage any underlying health conditions that could potentially affect the health of the bladder.

2. Strengthening the muscles of the pelvic floor can aid in the prevention of urinary incontinence and promote bladder health in general. Kegel exercises are a well-known and efficient method for accomplishing this.

3. It is important to restrict alcohol consumption as it can irritate the urethra and may also contribute to dehydration. If

possible, consume alcohol in moderation to promote bladder health.

4. Maintain an understanding of bladder health and UTI prevention through self-education. Understanding the contributing factors to urinary tract infections enables proactive risk reduction measures.

In Summary, The Attainment Of Bladder Bliss

A comprehensive strategy for bladder health is, in summary, critical for the prevention of urinary tract infections and the maintenance of general wellness. Consistent long-term habits, effective antibiotic use, bladder-friendly nutrition, and holistic wellness approaches all contribute to the attainment of bladder serenity.

By placing these health considerations as top priorities, individuals can adopt a preventative approach to bladder infections and maintain optimal urinary function for the duration of their lives.